A Supportive Guide to Overcoming
Life's Many Challenges

how to
cope when
everything's
gone to sh*t

Sam Cooper

HOW TO COPE WHEN EVERYTHING'S GONE TO SH*T

Text by Claire Chamberlain

An Hachette UK Company
www.hachette.co.uk

Vie Books, an imprint of Summersdale Publishers Ltd
Part of Octopus Publishing Group Limited
Carmelite House
50 Victoria Embankment
LONDON
EC4Y 0DZ
UK

www.summersdale.com

Printed and bound in China

ISBN: 978-1-83799-288-1

Substantial discounts on bulk quantities of Summersdale books are available to corporations, professional associations and other organizations. For details contact general enquiries: telephone: +44 (0) 1243 771107 or email: enquiries@summersdale.com.

Disclaimer
This book is not intended as a substitute for the medical advice of a doctor or physician. If you are experiencing problems with your physical or mental health, it is always best to follow the advice of a medical professional.

Have you enjoyed this book?
If so, why not write a review on your favourite website?

If you're interested in finding out more about our books, find us on Facebook at **Summersdale Publishers**, on Twitter at **@Summersdale** and on Instagram and TikTok at **@summersdalebooks** and get in touch. We'd love to hear from you!

Thanks very much for buying this Summersdale book.

www.summersdale.com

IT'S OK NOT TO BE OK

Good Advice and Kind Words For Positive Mental Well-Being

Claire Chamberlain

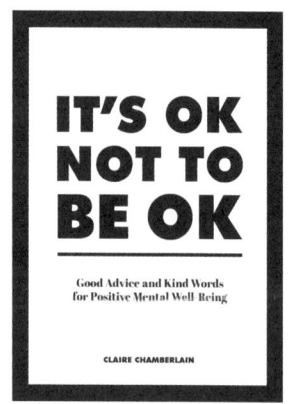

Hardback

ISBN: 978-1-78685-985-3

Into every life some rain must fall. Nobody is fine all the time, and if you're feeling down or struggling with serious problems, you're not alone. This clear and comforting guide is here to help you understand the mental health issues that can affect us all, and to help you look after your mind, body and soul. Touching on a range of topics, including anxiety, depression, loneliness, stress and self-esteem, this is a book for anyone and everyone who needs good advice, fresh ideas and kind words.

*Contents

4   Introduction

6   CHAPTER 1:
Why Does Everything Seem So Sh*t?

18   CHAPTER 2:
Coping With Life's Many Challenges

56   CHAPTER 3:
A Proactive Approach to Finding Calm

108   CHAPTER 4:
A Hopeful Future

142   CHAPTER 5:
Seeking Help

154   Conclusion

156   Resources

Introduction

Do you feel like life's gone to sh*t recently?

Do you dread checking the news in the morning (or even just opening your eyes) for fear of what you might be hit with? When your phone pings with an alert, do you feel your chest contract with panic, in case it's bad news? Are you struggling in your personal life, perhaps with financial difficulties, family conflict, grief, past trauma or relationship problems? Or do you just have a free-floating sense of anxiety – feelings of worry, fear or

foreboding – that you can't quite pin down to a particular cause, but that seems to be forever invading your mind?

If so, you've opened the right book. Within these pages, you'll find information on why you might be feeling the way you do, easy-to-implement tips on how to calm and clear your mind, and advice on regaining your sense of joy, hope and zest for life – even when times are tough.

Are you ready? Let's dive in together...

Why Does Everything Seem So Sh*t?

Sometimes, life can feel a bit sh*t. From personal crises to global fears, some days it's hard to filter out the bad news in order to embrace the good bits of life that feel as if they're out of reach (they're still there, we promise). This chapter takes a look at some of the reasons you might be feeling stressed, low, anxious or just plain sh*t – because before you can get back to living your best life, it can be helpful to understand and address what's preventing you.

You're not alone

If you feel like everything in your life is a bit sh*t right now, you're not alone. No, really – you aren't. Even people who look outwardly happy and shiny will experience feelings of insecurity, doubt and worry. And even if they're feeling shiny and happy right now, chances are they've had to navigate some sh*t times in the past. The point is, no one's life is perfect 24/7, even if it looks that way from the outside: all of us will have to navigate difficult, stressful and upsetting times, so always remember you're not alone.

The sliding scale of sh*t events

There are many situations, events or experiences that can make you feel a bit sh*t. These can be day-to-day annoyances (for example, your alarm not going off in the morning, a cancelled train or a spilled coffee); temporary stresses (such as struggling in an exam, financial worries or social media pressures); or huge life upheavals (such as bereavement or relationship breakdown).

It's a bit like a sliding scale of sh*t events: we can all probably identify times when

we've experienced things on both ends of the spectrum. The trouble is, when you have lots of these sh*t events going on at once, it can become overwhelming. And even if there are no big sh*t events in your life at the moment, lots of small or medium sh*t events piled up on top of each other can leave you feeling equally low, run-down and lacking in any sense of happiness or joy.

But don't despair – by learning the tools to strengthen your resilience and mindset, you can make it through even the toughest times.

Let's get personal

Personal struggles can often make it seem like everything's gone to sh*t. These include things like grief, bereavement, financial worries, job uncertainty, relationship breakdown, living with a chronic illness or coping with past trauma. If you're currently dealing with any of the above, it can feel incredibly lonely and isolating, but, if you feel able, there are ways you can help yourself, as well as external sources of support. We'll explore these options in greater depth in Chapter Two (from page 18).

Global triggers

Of course, it's not only personal issues that can leave us feeling stressed, anxious or overwhelmed. Events that are occurring on a global scale, such as the climate crisis, economic uncertainty and political division, are all serving to fuel an "anxiety epidemic". These large-scale concerns might be leaving you feeling overwhelmed and helpless and, of course, tackling them undoubtedly requires fundamental social and political change. But there are ways you can help to instigate positive change on a smaller scale, too, such as volunteering for a cause close to your heart (see page 98), which can help you feel more empowered and less overwhelmed.

Mental health 101

Some days you might receive bad news, see a triggering headline or have a disagreement with someone, and be left feeling anxious, sad or overwhelmed. However, on a different day, you might receive the same bad news, see the same headline or have the same disagreement, and be able to either brush it off, stay calm or find a solution. The difference? The state of your mental health.

Your mental health exists on a spectrum, which means it can shift up and down depending on many different factors at any given time. Some of these include:

* Your physical health
* Your support network

* Your environment

* Your lifestyle

When your mental health is good, you'll probably find you can cope better during challenges. But when something happens that affects your mental health for the worse, your positivity, resilience and ability to cope in the face of adversity will likely start to wobble. If your life feels sh*t right now, it could be that your mental health isn't so great. There's no shame in this: realizing there's a problem is often the first step to turning things round – and things can always turn around.

The truth about low mood

Partly due to the pressures of social media and its common "positive vibes only" rhetoric, we're often made to feel like there's something abnormal about feeling low, angry or upset.

But, in fact, the opposite is true: if you're currently facing difficult circumstances or life has just gotten seriously sh*t for you, these feelings are normal. It would be downright weird if you were skipping around happily in the face of such pressures.

Difficult feelings can be uncomfortable. But avoiding the truth of your life by

denying there's a problem or numbing yourself through other means will only add an extra layer of suffering. So, allow these feelings to exist. After all, everything you feel is valid, and acceptance is a vital first step.

However, if these feelings start to drift towards a sense of "emptiness", linger for more than a month, or are stopping you living your life, it could be a sign of something more going on, in which case, it's important to seek professional help. There's more information in Chapter Five (from page 142) on how to access support.

How this book can help

So far, we've explored some of the reasons why you might feel like everything's gone to sh*t right now. Perhaps your worries currently seem insurmountable, or you're feeling so low that you believe nothing you do will make a difference. But by identifying your fears and triggers, implementing steps to improve your mental health and learning how to seek out joy, you should see a marked improvement in your outlook – and your life!

Hopefully, the pages in this chapter have reassured you that if you're feeling sh*t right now, you're not alone. Not only are your feelings and concerns valid, but everyone feels this way sometimes, so try not to beat yourself up. The following chapters are going to help you address your worries and explore ways to take positive action, so if you do feel like everything's gone to sh*t, you might feel differently as you move through this book. Are you ready? Let's go!

Coping with Life's Many Challenges

When we consider the phrase "Everything's gone to sh*t", it's often associated with external issues – political chaos, the climate crisis or financial uncertainty, for example. But there are many internal, personal crises that can make you feel this way, too. In this chapter, we'll be exploring in greater depth the various issues that might be making you feel like crap, alongside ideas on how you might start to unravel and deal with these issues. Let's start figuring out how to get through this together...

First things first

Before we dive in, let's get something clear: there is no "right" way to feel. There's nothing wrong with you if you're struggling to cope with a challenging situation, so don't buy into thoughts that tell you otherwise. Going through a sh*t time is tough enough already, so try not to pile any more negativity onto your plate by telling yourself you need to do better. This isn't about changing anything that fundamentally makes you *you* (because you're perfect exactly as you are) – it's about learning to cope with difficult feelings, so that you can ultimately experience greater joy, happiness and freedom... all of which you deserve.

Understanding low mood

We all know what it's like to wake up feeling a bit sh*t: it's not quite sadness – you're just not your usual self. Perhaps you know the cause – maybe a recent break-up, pressure at work or worry about a family member has got you feeling flat. Or perhaps there's no clear reason as to why you feel low. If this is the case, remember that physical issues, such as tiredness, hormone fluctuations and mild illness, can affect your mood.

Your low mood might be trying to tell you something – perhaps that some things in your life right now are out of balance. Are you sleeping well? Eating a balanced diet?

Remembering to drink enough water each day? Try getting these basics back on track – sometimes a little self-care goes a long way and hopefully in a day or two you'll be feeling brighter.

If, however, your low mood is persistent and you just can't seem to shift it, or if you've begun to feel "empty", you may be suffering from symptoms of depression. If you've been feeling low or flat for a prolonged period of time, it's a good idea to make an appointment with your doctor, who will be able to offer confidential support.

Mental health vs mental health conditions

Knowing the difference between the root causes of mental health conditions and poor mental health is important, to ensure you get the right (and sufficient) support.

Mental health relates to your emotional and psychological well-being. If you're feeling pretty sh*t right now, it might be that something is affecting your well-being, causing it to be low. Where you are on the mental health spectrum at the moment will depend on lots of different factors, including the strength of your support network. While feeling a bit sh*t is, well... sh*t, you know it will

pass, especially if you're gentle with yourself during this difficult time.

A mental health condition, on the other hand (such as anxiety or obsessive compulsive disorder (OCD)), is thought to have genetic roots or be linked to brain chemistry. These usually require specialist professional treatment, such as talking therapy or medication, in addition to self-care. Sadly, chronic poor mental health can lead to conditions such as depression, so if you're feeling low, it's time to make a commitment to yourself and address it – your health and happiness matter.

Coping with stress

Exam stress, family stress, work stress, relationship stress – chances are we've all experienced stress at some point. Contrary to popular belief, stress is sometimes beneficial – "positive stress", or eustress, is a key driver for motivation and performance. Stress is uncomfortable, so it forces you to take action, get stuck in and do what you need to do to help alleviate the feeling.

It's only when stress becomes chronic (meaning you feel stressed all the time, without a specific trigger such as an exam or interview) that it can leave you feeling unable to cope. Is stress getting the better of you? It's important to try to find ways to cope, so you can protect your headspace. Ultimately, stress can make us feel a bit sh*t, but know there are strategies, such as breathwork (see page 61) and mindfulness techniques (see page 66), that can help.

Managing anxiety

Anxiety refers to feelings of dread, usually in relation to a future event (real or imagined). Most people experience it at some point (and yes, it can feel sh*t). Symptoms are often both mental and physical, and include excessive worrying, "butterflies" in your stomach and nausea. If your anxiety is getting out of hand (for example, if it's constant, your fears are out of proportion to the situation, or you avoid certain situations because of it), it might be worth visiting your doctor. You might be diagnosed with a specific disorder, such as social anxiety disorder, and will be offered appropriate support.

Panic attack tips

If you've ever experienced an abrupt onset of extreme fear, you might have had a panic attack. Symptoms often build quickly and can include a racing heart, shallow breath, trembling, sweating, chest pain and a fear you're going to collapse. While not physically dangerous, a panic attack can be intensely frightening. If you feel one happening, focus on breathing slowly and deeply. To lessen your chances of having an attack, it's important to work on lowering your stress levels. Daily breathing exercises, regular exercise and avoiding caffeine can all help.

Understanding OCD

OCD can be highly distressing and can creep up on you. It is characterized by obsessive thoughts that lead to repetitive compulsions, such as hand washing, checking locks or having to perform a task a certain number of times. While these ritualistic compulsions may initially seem to calm the obsessive thoughts, ultimately they can take over your life, causing significant distress and disruption. OCD can feel scary, but professional help is available and effective, so don't suffer in silence or in shame. Please also note that OCD can present itself in many different ways, so the best person to accurately diagnose you would be your doctor. Making an appointment with them is a great first step.

Here are some first steps you can take to help:

* Tell someone: Confiding in a loved one can offer support, and help to keep you accountable.

* Set a quitting date: Picking a date and writing this in your calendar or journal can add some structure to your recovery.

* Distract yourself: Taking up a hobby, completing exercise, or calling a friend during difficult moments can help to focus your mind elsewhere.

* Remove temptation: Making it harder to access your addiction means you'll be less likely to relapse.

* Seek professional help: Accessing support helps you to realize that you don't have to go it alone.

Managing feelings of anger

Anger has a pretty negative reputation, but perhaps not deservedly so. Remember, anger is a perfectly healthy emotion in the face of frustration, deceit or inequality. If you feel that you or someone you care about has been wronged, it's natural to feel angry about it. Used constructively, it can steer us to respond assertively – anger is a key emotion that compels us to act in ways that we sometimes need to.

However, if you notice outbursts of rage (either verbal or physical) creeping up regularly, it can have very negative consequences.

Try these tips to help you get those outbursts under control:

* Give yourself a cooling off "time out", so you can collect your thoughts and respond calmly a little later, rather than reacting aggressively in the moment.

* Become mindful of your body and your surroundings: shifting the focus of your attention can help you stay grounded.

* Take a few deep breaths. This is a tried-and-tested anger management tip for good reason: taking deep, relaxed breaths helps to engage the parasympathetic nervous system (which signals your body to relax), in turn switching off other physical anger symptoms, such as elevated heart rate and tensed muscles.

Handling conflict

Wherever it arises – be it at work, home, with a friend or a total stranger – conflict is always stressful. If you find yourself caught up in a confrontation, try to stay calm. Conflict doesn't have to become argumentative if you don't let it – take a deep breath, which will give you a moment's pause and a greater chance to respond thoughtfully rather than react violently. Beginning sentences with "I feel…" (e.g. "I feel I'm taking on the majority of the workload", instead of, "You always leave everything to me… you're so lazy") can help to remove overt accusations, keeping things constructive.

Managing low self-esteem

Low self-esteem can stem from lots of different things, such as stressful life events or comparing ourselves to others. Internalizing harmful remarks, even if they were said by someone whose opinion we shouldn't pay attention to (like a childhood bully), can shape the way we view ourselves. If you have low self-esteem, you might feel stuck in your head a lot, so mindfulness can help. By living in the moment without self-judgement, you'll feel free to cast off unhelpful self-perceptions and get on with living your life fully. If low self-esteem is affecting the way you live your life, make an appointment with your doctor for professional support and advice.

Coping with failure and rejection

Rejection and failure hurt. Like, really hurt. Whether the rejection is from a partner, friend or someone else, or whether you haven't made the grade in an exam or your job application got rejected, for instance, feeling like something external to you is saying "You're not good enough" can really knock your self-worth. But rejection is a common human experience (however sh*t it feels). In fact, everyone will feel like a failure at some point, so learning to cope (and even thrive afterwards) is key.

The first step involves taking time to grieve the lost opportunity or partnership. It hurts because it mattered, so pretending it didn't won't help. If you feel able, leaning into that hurt can offer a much-needed release (hint: having a good cry is cathartic). Don't berate yourself, though: self-kindness is vital here. Treat yourself the way you would a friend who is dealing with rejection or failure: with utmost compassion. After processing the pain, it's time to build resilience (there's no set timeline here, just whenever you feel ready). Focus on what you can learn from the experience and remind yourself that whatever you feel you've lost wasn't meant for you: better experiences, opportunities and relationships might be just around the corner.

Dealing with change

While change can be a positive thing, signalling opportunities for growth, it can also feel scary. After all, change often goes hand in hand with uncertainty, which by its very nature can be anxiety inducing. So, if you're going through a big life change right now, such as moving to a new area or leaving a long-term relationship or job, go easy on yourself. Even though it's exciting, recognize and accept the fact that experiencing nerves, worry and fear are all perfectly normal reactions, too (sh*t, yes, but normal).

If your fear of change is becoming a problem (stopping you from moving forward, taking any chances or going for something that deep down you really want to do, for instance), grab your journal, notebook or a piece of paper, and write down a list of all the things you might gain from embracing the big change. Next, write down how your life might look one year from now if you take that leap of faith. These simple writing exercises can help you see the positives in taking that first brave step. Because yes, embracing change takes courage, but you can do it.

Handling social media pressure

Social media can be inspiring... but it's important to recognize its dark side, too. If you're constantly scrolling through other people's online lives, in what can be a never-ending conveyor belt of happy faces, exotic adventures, dream interiors and "perfect" bodies, there's the potential for your own life to suddenly feel sh*t in comparison. If this sounds familiar, remember: people only post highlights – and no one's life is filled with highlights 24/7. It's your social feed, so feel free to curate it to suit you: don't follow people who make you feel sh*t... unfollow, block and mute at will!

Balancing work and life

In this "always on" society, where bosses or colleagues can contact you via phone or email any hour of the day, the line between work and home has become increasingly blurred. If you feel like your work-life balance is seriously out of kilter and is leaving you stressed and burned out, it's time to set boundaries. Get clear on your work hours, turn off access to work emails on your personal phone, take your lunch breaks and start getting comfortable communicating with your boss to let them know if you're feeling overwhelmed. Feeling "on" 24/7 is sh*t, so try to prioritize finding and maintaining that all-important balance.

Managing financial difficulties

Money worries are a common mental health trigger. Unemployment, having to manage an irregular income and constantly having to pay for things can be highly stressful, and overdrafts, unpaid bills and maxed-out credit cards can lead to sleepless nights. Debt often feels overwhelming and like yet more sh*t to deal with, but remember, there are measures you can take to start regaining control. Seeking advice from a financial support charity is a great place to start, or call your bank to find out what your options are. Setting yourself a daily or weekly budget or focusing on paying off one debt first are also good steps to reducing your stress levels.

Addressing relationship problems

If you and your partner are currently experiencing difficulties, opening up is key. Do you think your partner knows how you're feeling? Often, problems and resentment can build through lack of communication (and, yes, we know that sh*t can be hard). Can you set aside time to talk through how you're feeling? Remember to listen to your partner, too – their experience and interpretation is as equally valid as yours. Collaboration and respect are vital in any relationship, as is honouring each other's boundaries. Are your differences worth working through together?

Coping with grief and bereavement

The loss of someone or something important to you, such as a loved one or pet, a dream job or opportunity will be painful. Really, deeply, heavily painful. It can feel endless and, while this all-consuming sadness *will* pass, remember there's no set timeline, so give yourself space to grieve. Also remember, there is no right or wrong way to grieve – it's a personal experience. You might feel sadness, anger, regret – let it all come through and try not to suppress anything.

Allow yourself to feel your emotions, however difficult it can be, rather than bottling your grief up. Try not to be afraid

to ask for support – if you've lost a loved one, there are bereavement charities with listening services that can help. If you feel able, talk to those around you; sharing memories, stories, experiences and insights is not only a great way to process grief, but it can also be a powerful bonding experience, during which you might form a deeper connection with others.

Finally, it might be a cliché, but time is a great healer, so allow yourself plenty of it, and don't expect too much of yourself too soon. Moments of joy will begin to creep through once more, probably when you least expect it, so hang in there.

Responding to global injustices

Cultural, political and social inequality, extreme poverty, overt and systemic racism, sexism and violence against women... the list of widespread global injustices goes on and on. If you're struggling with feelings of helplessness, grief or anger in the face of such inequality, channelling this into action, such as joining protest groups or marches, can be the most empowering and effective form of resistance to systemic abuse and discrimination.

However, activism itself can take its toll on your mental health, too. From pages 96 to 107, we'll take a look at ways to get involved

with activism and how it can help you to stay hopeful for the future. And once you get stuck in (or if you're currently involved in activism), looking after your mental health is key. Make sure you take time each week to switch off from the important work and have a little downtime: relax, exercise, watch your favourite show, meditate, do something that sparks joy, and spend time noticing and expressing gratitude for the good things in life, too. Try not to feel guilty for taking this time out – you're best positioned to make a difference in the world when you're at your best yourself.

Coping with eco-anxiety

Eco-anxiety springs from feelings of uncertainty and frustration in relation to climate change. It's easy to slip into a state of helplessness, but channelling your climate grief into climate action can help both the planet and your own mental health. This might be by making changes to your personal behaviour in order to live in a more environmentally friendly way (for example, by composting food waste, growing bee-friendly plants or using a reusable bag), or by joining activist groups or climate support networks. The key is to lessen the feelings of anxiety by using it to fuel proactive change. If you're really struggling, cognitive behavioural therapy (CBT) can be useful for all forms of anxiety.

Write down your worries

If you feel like everything's gone to sh*t, writing down your worries can help. This is especially true if you tend to experience free-floating anxiety or if you feel overwhelmed by what's going on for you. Write down everything that's concerning you – regardless of how "big" or "small" they may seem. Seeing things in black and white can sometimes help you to rationalize them. Is there anything you can easily address, such as life admin hanging over your head, or a difficult phone call you could get out of the way? Are there things that are outside of your power? Crossing them off the list can be a powerfully symbolic way of letting go.

Remove everyday triggers

It might sound obvious, but steering clear of the things that worry, upset or enrage you, or that trigger traumatic memories, can help you feel calmer. Of course, this isn't always possible (the anniversary of a loved one's death will always come around, or you might have to liaise with that passive-aggressive colleague), but are there any sources of irritation or upset that you could just avoid? For example, can you mute triggering people on social media, or switch off news notifications on your phone? Removing triggers from your day-to-day life can leave your mind feeling clearer.

Focus on what you can control

There are plenty of things outside your control: the traffic, the weather, how someone responds to your email, an employer not shortlisting you for an interview. So, try to forget about these things. Instead, focus on what you *can* control. Traffic's bad? Try listening to a podcast to turn this "dead time" into "me time". It starts raining? Why not duck into a nearby coffee shop for a welcome recharge? Someone takes something the wrong way? Know that you're only in control of your intent, not other people's interpretations. Didn't get your dream job? How might you hone your CV or upskill to give yourself the best shot next time? Always take accountability where you can and forget all the other sh*t.

Reshape your mindset

So often, the way we view ourselves and the world comes down to mindset. If you have a negative mindset, you'll tend to focus on the downside and struggle to see the good things right in front of you. If you have a positive mindset, you'll be able to seek out small joys even in challenging circumstances. The good news is, mindset isn't fixed. By working on your mindset, outlook and resilience, harnessing some of the tips in Chapter Three (from page 56), you'll probably find that life starts to feel more exciting and joyful – even if your external circumstances haven't changed at all.

Get proactive!

There's a saying, "Worry is like a rocking chair: it gives you something to do, but doesn't get you anywhere." If you feel like worries are going round and round in your head, but nothing's changing, maybe it's time to get proactive. Choose a problem that's been bothering you for some time. What steps might you be able to take to find a solution? Is there someone you could speak to, or a campaign you could join, or a letter you could write, or a petition you could sign? Taking action, however small you may think it is, can help you to feel better, as you'll be channelling your concern into positive steps that will make a difference. Discover more proactive steps you can take to find calm in Chapter Three, over the page!

A Proactive Approach to Finding Calm

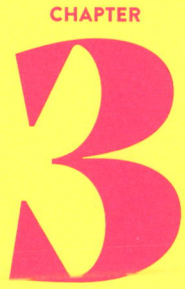

So far, we've delved into the many reasons why you might feel like everything's gone to sh*t. Understanding what's going on for you is important, but when it comes to managing and improving your mental health, the next step is to change your mindset, build your resilience and be kind to yourself (a more radical idea than you might think!). This chapter details a host of tips to help you actively seek happiness and calm.

Your mental health matters

Before we delve into proactively inviting calm, happiness and growth into our lives, let's first clarify why mental health matters. Perhaps you don't believe yours does – or you don't believe you deserve happiness for some reason – or maybe you've simply never thought about it before. The fact is, your mental health matters immensely: cultivating good mental health will positively influence pretty much every aspect of your life, from your personal happiness and ability to handle stress, to your resilience in the face of challenges, relationships and interactions, physical health and even professional and career development.

The importance of accountability

If you're going to commit to your own healing, then you're going to have to try to get comfortable with being accountable for your own growth, mindset and mental health – in the face of whatever life throws at you. Because unfortunately sh*t will happen in your life (as it happens in everyone's life at some point), but you don't have to let these things define you.

Think for a moment of someone whose mindset inspires you – it might be a celebrity, an inspirational speaker or someone you know personally. Has this person sailed through life, without encountering any challenges, setbacks or trauma? Unlikely. Instead, they've

probably faced their problems with courage, determination, dignity and a positive mindset – and you can learn to do this, too.

Becoming accountable for your own life means not blaming others – or circumstances – when things go wrong (and sometimes they do go spectacularly wrong!). It means working on your resilience, focusing on what you can control, and remaining as hopeful, positive and determined as you can in the face of adversity. The late Dame Deborah James spoke of having "rebellious hope", which is a profoundly positive way to face adversity. How can you bring more rebellious hope into your own life?

How to build resilience

We've talked a fair amount about resilience so far – but what exactly is it? In a nutshell, your resilience refers to how well you withstand or recover from the sh*t life throws at you. There are some key things that can help you strengthen your resilience: self-awareness (which includes accountability in tough times), mindfulness, self-care techniques, a sense of purpose, and your connection with others. Check out how to harness the power of your breath (page 61), go for a mindful walk (page 68), or develop a meditation routine (page 72), to instill a greater sense of positivity and calm in your life.

Coping with loneliness

Whether you haven't found a network of friends yet or you're currently spending lots of time alone, loneliness sucks. But never forget: if you're currently lonely, it *doesn't* mean there's something wrong with you. You're brilliant, even if you don't have people to share your wonderfulness with right now. Have a go at building a connection with someone – it could be a colleague you'd like to get to know better outside of work, a fellow parent at the school gates or a friend you've lost contact with. A quick chat, message or voice note is often all it takes. And even though feeling lonely can be a bit sh*t, remember your own company is also something to be treasured.

Combatting disordered eating

While eating disorders refer to mental health conditions that can be diagnosed with a specific set of criteria, such as anorexia nervosa, disordered eating is a descriptive term that refers to problems with food that fall outside of these criteria.

Disordered eating can still be serious and upsetting and can include behaviours such as making rigid rules about food (such as only being able to eat at certain times of day), comfort eating, binge eating and meal

skipping. All of these can potentially lead to rapid fluctuations in weight, which can be harmful to your health.

In the short term, growing an awareness of your body's needs and dietary preferences, and paying attention to hunger cues can help. But if you think you have a problem with eating, opening up to a professional who can offer confidential support and guidance is key, so make an appointment with your doctor. Yes, speaking openly about your eating habits might be difficult, but you don't have to go through this alone.

Understanding addiction

Most of us have probably tried taking the edge off a painful, difficult or sh*tty experience by numbing it with something. People attempt to numb pain with all manner of things: food, sugar, shopping, alcohol... even social media scrolling. The problems start when numbing becomes a chronic and compulsive habit.

Addiction is a mental health condition, but sadly there is still often huge stigma attached to it. If you feel like you've lost control of a habit, or that it's getting to the point of becoming dangerous and you're struggling, don't feel ashamed.

Take deep breaths

When you're anxious or stressed, you might notice your breathing becomes shallow and rapid. Research has shown that taking control of your breathing can help you regain a sense of calm. Deep breathing is also a wonderful ritual to incorporate into your mornings, helping you feel grounded and ready for the day ahead. When you wake up, take a moment to perform five slow, deep breaths, inhaling for a count of six and exhaling for a count of six, both through your nose. Deep breathing activates your parasympathetic nervous system, which tells your brain that you're safe, slows your heart rate and lowers cortisol levels (the primary stress hormone). Repeat throughout the day to help counteract some of those negative emotions.

You deserve to feel calm

If you don't believe you deserve happiness or peace, let's take a moment to shut that negative thinking down. Whatever's happened in your life, you deserve to feel good. Poor mental health can eventually make you feel undeserving of joy and contentment – but this can actually create unconscious resistance to positive change, resulting in self-sabotage. So yes, there may be a whole lot of sh*t in your past – loss, trauma, shame, regret or anger, maybe – but to move on, you need to be gentle with yourself and truly believe that you deserve peace, joy, happiness, love... all the good stuff!

Make time for relaxation

What with work, study, commuting, general responsibilities and all that other sh*t, it's no wonder many of us feel we don't have time for self-care. But don't demote yourself to the bottom of your to-do list! Self-care will boost your mental health, mindset and resilience, so it's vital if you want to be able to keep going for everything (and everyone!) else in your life. If time's tight, make use of "fringe" hours, such as early mornings or lunch breaks. Think also about times where you're simply waiting – for a train or for food to cook, for example. Reclaim these moments for yourself!

Getting clear on self-care

Before we dive into all things self-care, we need to clear up what self-care means. The biggest thing to understand is that self-care absolutely doesn't mean denying difficult or upsetting feelings. It's not about stepping into a candlelit bath, plastering a smile on your face and telling yourself everything's great when, deep down, you feel like sh*t. Instead, it's about being kind to yourself when times are good *and* bad, in order to build resilience and help you deal with hard times. It refers to any deliberate act that protects and improves your physical, mental and emotional health, such as practising mindfulness, making time for meditation and developing a healthy sleep routine.

Self-care vs damage control

Are you guilty of turning to self-care as a last resort, once your mental health has already plummeted? You're not alone – many of us attempt to use self-care as some kind of desperate damage control once things already feel sh*t. But it's much harder to navigate difficult feelings and emotions when you're already engulfed by them. Establishing a solid self-care regime *before* times of crisis is far more helpful, enabling you to navigate and even sidestep low moments. Making self-care a daily habit is a truly nurturing and life-affirming step – are you ready to commit to yourself?

Develop a mindfulness routine

If you want to feel like you're really, truly, deeply living your life (as opposed to being so stuck in your head that you miss the day-to-day goings-on around you), then mindfulness is a must.

Yes, it's been a buzzword for a long time now, but with good reason: practise it daily and it can help with stress, anxiety and even depression, by drawing you out of your thoughts and into the present moment. Because that's all mindfulness is: becoming consciously aware of the present moment, without judgement or without trying to

change anything. It's a way of becoming connected to the "right now" of life.

While it sounds simple enough, it can take a little practice – especially if you're used to being caught up in myriad thoughts, worries and fears.

Start with just 5 minutes a day, drawing your attention away from your thoughts and out into the world around you. Focus on each sense in turn: what can you see, feel, hear, smell, taste? When thoughts arise that distract you (and trust me, they will), simply draw your attention back to the present moment. In time, mindfulness can help you become comfortable during life's sh*t moments.

Go for a mindful walk

Even a short walk of 10 to 15 minutes can be enough to reset your busy mind. But how often have you gone out to give yourself some headspace, only to find you spend the whole time so caught up in worries that you miss everything en route? This is where mindfulness techniques can help. Consciously taking notice of everything around you – from the birdsong, to the breeze on your face, to the cars driving by, to the feel of your feet connecting with the path – will help to keep you grounded in the moment, so you truly get a break from your thoughts. Try taking a daily mindful walk to clear your head, setting yourself up to better cope with the sh*t life throws at you.

Start journalling

Writing can be both cathartic and revealing: you might start scribbling on one subject, but then find yourself opening up about some hidden truth or problem. This is why journalling can be so eye-opening and healing. You don't need a fancy journal to get started – any old notebook will do. Try a few minutes of "stream of consciousness" writing – just writing whatever comes into your head. It might be what you can see in front of you, or something that happened that day – just keep the words flowing: you might be surprised by what ends up on the page. Once all the sh*t is out of your head and onto the page, you're likely to feel a lot calmer.

The transformative power of gratitude

If you could take a magic potion each day that promised to deepen your happiness, help you handle adversity, strengthen your relationships, improve your sleep quality, lift your mood and boost your immunity, AND it had no adverse side effects (plus to top it off, it was free!), would you take it? Well, guess what? Expressing gratitude on a daily basis has been proven to do all of the above!

Try keeping a daily gratitude journal, in which you write down three things you're grateful for every day. Or maybe share what

you're grateful for with your partner, friends or family at the end of each day.

It doesn't have to be big things, either – being grateful for a beautiful sunrise, your hot cup of coffee, the chance to read a few pages of your book, the daisies brightening up the garden, or your partner cooking dinner for you are all great examples of small things that might brighten your day. By actively encouraging your mind to seek out things it appreciates, you start to hardwire your brain to look out for the positives in life, thereby changing your overall mindset and outlook. What might you feel grateful for today?

Try meditation

Don't have time to meditate? Then you'd probably benefit from it! Yes, you lead a full-on life – but might you be able to find just 5 or 10 minutes each day to sit quietly in meditation?

Carving out this time will do wonders for your well-being, with studies showing a regular meditation practice can result in reduced stress, lessened anxiety and enhanced self-awareness (all of those good things that help to build resilience, improve mindset and instill calm). Basically, meditation is a technique we can use to help us find our calm before, during, or after a day of dealing with sh*t.

Meditation might sound spiritual (and indeed, it forms a basis of many spiritual

practices), but when it comes down to it, it's simply focused attention without judgement.

To give it a go, ensure you're in a quiet place and sit comfortably. There are many ways to meditate, but one of the simplest is to pay attention to your breath. Close your eyes, then follow each inhale and exhale, without trying to change your breathing pattern. Your mind will probably wander. This is normal: as soon as you notice your attention has shifted, simply acknowledge the thought, then draw your attention back to your breath. If you're struggling to get started, guided meditations are great – access them online or via a meditation app.

Practise yoga

A yoga practice doesn't have to take up hours each day to be effective: simply starting each day with a few minutes of gentle, conscious stretching can be enough to clear your mind, reduce stress and improve your mindset (even researchers agree this could be the case, with studies showing that yoga can reduce stress, anxiety, depression and chronic pain, and can enhance the overall quality of your life). Try a few gentle postures to get you started, such as downward-facing dog, forward fold and child's pose, or a few gentle sun salutations. If you're unfamiliar with yoga, finding a local class is a great idea to ensure you do the poses correctly, or there are lots of online tutorials available.

Join a class

Is there something you've always fancied trying your hand at but have never had the confidence to do? Then why not gently push yourself out of your comfort zone and sign up for a class? Learning a new skill can help dig you out of a rut (perfect if you've begun to think life's a bit sh*t), plus it proves to you you're capable of growth and change, which in turn boosts confidence and self-esteem. From art classes, jewellery making and learning a new language, to circus skills and rock climbing, there's bound to be something that sparks your interest.

Invest time in hobbies

It's not just about taking up new skills and hobbies – what about the things you already know you love doing? Do you still make time for them regularly? When we're feeling overwhelmed, low, stressed or anxious, we often let our favourite hobbies and activities slide – especially when sh*t gets hectic. But carving out time for something you love can help you to stay mindful (as it focuses your attention on the present moment) and can spark feelings of joy, fulfilment and purpose. What have you always loved doing? Baking? Running? Crafting? Dancing? Playing a sport? Maybe it's time to reignite the passion.

Connect with your inner child

Have you ever noticed how absorbed children get when they play – how those building blocks receive 100 per cent of their concentration; how those toys come to life for them; how the floor really *is* lava? As adults, we've forgotten the powerfully absorbing effects of play. And there are other benefits, too: play stimulates the imagination, helps with problem-solving, boosts creativity and releases stress. So, get yourself a skipping rope, do some mindful colouring, balance along a fallen tree – discover childlike joy again! It will promote well-being and calm your mind.

Seek out joy

Joyful moments don't always jump out in front of you, waving frantically to get your attention. Generally, if you want to experience more joy, happiness and positivity in life, you have to go searching for it. You need to try putting yourself in situations that will make you feel happy, and stay present and mindful in all the "ordinary" day-to-day moments. This way, you'll be more able to spot those precious moments of joy, beauty and connection.

Things like stepping outside and putting your feet in the grass while you drink your coffee, pausing to listen to the birds as you walk outside, taking a photo of that flower growing through a crack in the pavement, calling a friend for a spontaneous catch-up, hugging a loved one, cooking an exciting new recipe for dinner, taking a breakfast picnic on a hike, heading out super early to catch the sunrise, patting a cute dog... All these small, simple and yet transformative moments are out there, waiting for you to notice them, interact with them and create them. So go on – seek them out!

Meet up with friends

One of the simplest things you can do to release stress, promote well-being and actively induce a calmer state of mind is to spend time with a friend or two. You don't have to do anything fancy: simply hanging out, chatting, laughing and reminiscing can do wonders for both your mental and physical health. Everyone's got sh*t going on, so carving out time together might be tricky, but human connection is important, and getting a regular date in the diary will give you something to look forward to.

Do exercise you love

Yes, exercise is great at improving your physical health, but did you know it's amazing for your mind, too? Exercise is a great way to tackle those "everything's gone to sh*t" feelings, by flooding your body with endorphins (the feel-good hormones). And there's more: you don't need to commit to running a marathon to reap these mental health rewards – simply moving a little every day is a brilliant start. So, try taking the stairs instead of the elevator, cycle instead of drive, take a short daily walk or dance around the kitchen while you wait for the kettle to boil – anything that gets your heart racing will equal a happier, healthier you!

Try cold-water therapy

It might sound horrifying, but don't dismiss a cold-water dip: it's an amazing way to get an instant mood boost and can leave your mind feeling calm afterwards. Cold-water enthusiasts extoll the virtues of wild swimming in the sea, rivers and lakes, but you can get a similar effect from a cool shower. If you're going to get your cold kicks in the wild, safety is paramount: make sure you're fully prepared, follow safety guidelines and never swim alone. Even if you opt for the icy shower option, be mindful of health conditions, especially relating to the heart. (Ensure you consult your doctor if you have concerns.)

Stay hydrated

Staying hydrated is vital for your physical health, but being properly hydrated can boost your mood, too. Not only does drinking water help you stay mentally focused, but it can even stave off anxiety and fatigue. Feeling low? Try drinking a glass of water. (OK, it might not be the only answer, but trying certainly won't do any harm, and drinking water will ensure you're fully hydrated and better able to function with all the day-to-day sh*t.) It's recommended you drink between six and eight glasses a day. If plain water doesn't float your boat, try adding lime wedges, cucumber slices or berries for flavour – and don't forget juices, herbal teas, tea, coffee and even soup all count towards your hydration.

Eat to fuel your body

Healthy eating is all about fuelling yourself with foods that make you feel happy, calm and alert. Some of the best brain-boosting foods that have been shown to ease anxiety include products rich in GABA (gamma-aminobutyric acid, which is known to calm the nervous system). Good examples of these are broccoli, brown rice, lentils, bananas and spinach. Foods high in B vitamins (which help us store and use energy from protein and carbohydrates), such as leafy greens, salmon and eggs, can also improve mental health, by helping to regulate mood. Eating healthily is absolutely not about restricting or dieting, so don't forget the odd treat, too (cake, anyone?).

Avoid too much alcohol

Feel like everything's gone to sh*t? If you drink alcohol, it's important to remember that it's a depressant, so it's probably not helping matters. Obviously enjoying the odd glass or two a few times a week isn't a problem, but if you're drinking often, or in large quantities, it's going to start placing a strain on both your mind and body. Might you need to start cutting back? We'd all benefit from sticking to the weekly recommendations of 14 units a week (roughly six medium glasses of wine) or less, with at least two consecutive alcohol-free days.

Spend more time in nature

If you're feeling low, stressed or anxious and you spend lots of your time indoors or in an urban environment, you might be suffering from nature-deficit disorder. While not a medical diagnosis, the term seeks to name a very real crisis that affects many people – a disconnect from the natural world – with symptoms including emotional illness and attention difficulties. The solution? Spending more "mindful time in nature", according to Richard Louv, the author who coined the term.

Indeed, spending time in the natural world comes with a host of well-documented mental health benefits. Many studies show

it can do everything from boosting your mood and reducing stress, to easing anxiety and depression.

The Japanese tradition of *shinrin-yoku* (forest bathing) is now being widely adopted by Western cultures in an effort to rebalance our lives. The practice simply involves immersion in nature, by walking slowly through (or sitting quietly in) a forest or woodland and experiencing it with all of your senses. Even sitting outside with your feet in the grass can help you feel more grounded, or invest in some houseplants to bring a little of the outside in – you might be amazed at how calming it can feel.

Get your hands dirty

With studies showing gardening as a great way to reduce stress, increase self-esteem and promote calm, flexing your green fingers can be a wonderful mood-booster. What's more, soil can actually make you happy (which sounds wild, but it's true!). Soil contains the bacteria Mycobacterium vaccae, which gets absorbed through the skin when gardening and triggers the release of serotonin (the happy hormone) in the brain. Put simply, soil is good sh*t! You don't need an allotment or garden to reap the benefits – if you don't have access to outside space, planting a window box of herbs, chillies or tomato plants is a great way to get your hands dirty, too.

Be more *wabi sabi*

Life is rarely perfect, yet often we expect it to be. We assume happiness should be our default setting, so resist difficult experiences and emotions – experiences and emotions that are all part of being human. But what might happen if we embraced all of it – all the mess, imperfection and uncertainty of our lives? Accepting the bad parts as well as the good? With the expectation of perfection removed, we might feel a little more free and better able to cope when things go wrong. This is a bit like the Japanese aesthetic of *wabi sabi*, which acknowledges three truths: nothing lasts, nothing is finished and nothing is perfect. If we can be a bit more *wabi sabi*, and embrace and accept the imperfection in things, we can learn to live life to the full, even when everything's gone to sh*t.

Curl up with a page-turner

Honestly, who doesn't love losing themselves in the pages of a good book whenever life feels sh*t? And with good reason! Reading is comforting, anxiety relieving and can immerse us in a world different than our own, and science proves it. Researchers have found getting lost in the pages of a book actually lowers stress levels, due to the fact that getting caught up in an absorbing storyline allows you to shut out real life, even if it's just for a little while. The ultimate escapism! Have you noticed how your mind has become focused on this page, even, blocking out the sh*t going on beyond this book?

Treat yourself

Have you ever brightened a friend's day with a small treat – a bunch of flowers, a bar of chocolate, a card to let them know you're thinking of them? If you're feeling sh*t and your day could do with a boost, there's no need to wait for someone else to do it for you! Treat yourself to a little pick-me-up. It doesn't have to be expensive – a nice coffee, a book from the second-hand store or a cupcake from the bakery are all ways to give your own day a little lift. You could even simply cook yourself your favourite meal. Start being a friend to yourself. You deserve it!

Rest and recharge

Sometimes, despite feeling totally rubbish, you might be able to plaster a smile across your face, brave the world and get sh*t done. If today is not one of those days, that's OK. If your mental health is in a bad place and you're feeling down, give yourself a break and allow yourself a much-needed duvet day, so that you can rest. You could even plan a recharge day into your schedule after a busy period: sleep, rest, read, have a hot drink, curl up on the sofa and binge your favourite series. Do whatever you need to recuperate. Tomorrow is a fresh start, so banish the guilt and give yourself permission to rest.

Have a power nap

Oh, the joy of an afternoon nap! What better way to recharge and find a sense of calm than to snuggle under the covers and enjoy 20 minutes of shut-eye? What's more, research shows that afterwards, you may find you have better concentration and memory recall, as well as improved alertness. So bedding down in your afternoon break is a win-win, hopefully leaving you feeling more productive later in the day. Try not to nap after 4 p.m., as this could disrupt your night-time sleep, and keep your nap short but sweet – 20 to 25 minutes is best, so you don't feel too groggy afterwards. If you're in an office or workplace and naps aren't exactly an option, try taking regular screen breaks, instead. The mini-rest will help you deal with any incoming sh*t later in the day.

Go on a social media detox

Yes, social media keeps you connected, but is this constant connectivity negatively affecting your mental health? Social media can be great, but it also has the capacity to make you feel sh*t, especially if you feel pressured to constantly create content, you're caught up in a comparison cycle, or endless #ads from influencers are starting to grate your nerves. Research shows a social media detox (anything from a few days to a few months) can help to reduce anxiety levels, improve sleep patterns, boost mental well-being and lessen stress. Regularly taking some time away from social media can help you protect your headspace, prioritizing your calm.

Get enough sleep

With studies showing that regular poor sleep can result in flattened emotional responses, it's no wonder you feel like everything's gone to sh*t if you're not getting enough rest. Adults need roughly 8 hours of sleep each night, but you may need to spend longer in bed to achieve this – perhaps 9 hours. Can't seem to nod off? Establishing a sleep routine (going to bed and getting up at the same time each day), avoiding screens in the hour before bed, and ensuring your sleep environment is comfortable and quiet (ear plugs and blackout blinds can be lifesavers in urban areas) might help.

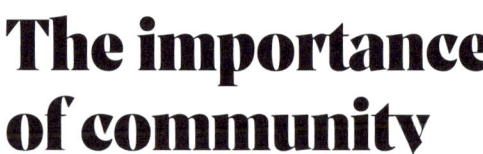

The importance of community

Community is so important because it gives us a sense of belonging and connection. Communities can be large or small – your town or city is a community, for example, but so are the smaller networks you belong to, such as your workplace, college, clubs, teams or activist groups. Our communities give us the chance to come together over shared values and passions, or to discuss our fears and concerns.

If you're feeling sh*t because of broader issues – whether it's a local community concern or the wider state of the world –

taking positive action as part of your wider community can be the best bet for your mental health.

If there's something bothering you, now's the time to stand up, step in and help make a difference. Doing something for others – whether that's within your local community or helping to campaign for global change – will help you feel more empowered, which in turn can boost your self-esteem and improve your mental health. The following tips should give you some ideas on how to get started, such as volunteering for a cause close to your heart (see page 98), or joining a protest (see page 106).

Volunteer for a good cause

Feel like the world's gone to sh*t? It might be because you're stuck in your own head, playing worst-case scenarios over and over, or only seeing the negatives in life. One thing that can help is actively looking for the good: good people, valuable projects and meaningful causes.

There are lots of people out there working to make positive, impactful change. And while simply seeking them out and showing appreciation for their work is great, the most rewarding thing to do is to join them! Research shows those who spend time volunteering often feel a strong sense of purpose, as well as increased happiness and confidence.

Is there a project, cause or campaign you care about that you could volunteer for? There are so many possibilities, including becoming a dementia befriender, volunteering at an animal sanctuary, supporting children's reading at a local primary school, getting involved in a climate change group's campaigning, doing local litter picking, getting stuck into a community gardening project, making posters, or donating clothes or toiletries.

Check out community noticeboards or online groups to see where you can lend a hand. Even if you can only spare an hour a week, it will be time well spent, and knowing you're helping to make the world a little less sh*t is the best way to feel like you're taking back control and creating positive change.

Simply do a good turn

Helping others doesn't have to be a big deal or cost you any money. Simply committing to helping those around you when you are able can make a huge difference to their lives – and will make you feel better, too! Offering to do things such as babysit for a friend, walk a neighbour's dog, pop to the shops for your parent or help a relative set up their new gadget are relatively small gestures that can go a long way. Who do you know who might need a hand? Life's a little less sh*t when everyone helps each other out.

Get involved with fundraising

From races to raffles, sponsored silences to skydives, football tournaments to fancy dress days, raising money for a cause close to your heart is a brilliant way to give something back and feel a sense of pride. It's also a great way to add meaning and purpose to an activity or challenge, and if you contact your chosen charity to let them know what you're doing, you'll become part of their fundraising team, which will add a real sense of community and connection to your efforts. Online sponsorship sites and crowdfunding means fundraising can be super straightforward – so pick your cause and start giving them (and yourself!) a boost.

Reach out to someone who's lonely

Let's face it: feeling lonely is sh*t. It's something we've probably all experienced at some point, and that sense of isolation and aloneness can be deeply painful. Let's just take a moment here to reassure you that, if you're feeling lonely right now and think there must be something wrong with you, there is nothing the matter with you.

Reaching out to others who might be feeling lonely can not only help them, but it can also deepen our own sense of connection.

Check out local groups and classes to help you connect with new, like-minded people – there will be loads out there, from book clubs to sports teams, so pick something

that appeals to you. And don't forget to use online resources, too: friend-finding services, such as Bumble For Friends, can be a great way to connect with others.

Statistics show that social isolation increases with age and, in the UK alone, some 1.4 million elderly people report feeling lonely, according to a report conducted by Age UK. Do you have an elderly neighbour you can check in on? Stopping for a chat if you see them out and about might make their day, or maybe you could offer to help them with their shopping, or invite them round for a cup of tea once in a while.

Isolation feels horrible and can be a leading cause of depression. Making time for a lonely person might seem a small thing to you, but it could be everything to them – and who knows, your budding new friendship might bloom into something wonderful and lifelong!

Sign a petition

Sometimes, doing something positive and proactive can take as little as a minute – the time it takes to write your name on an online petition and click "add". If you're feeling stressed or low because of a particular issue, adding your name to (or even starting) a petition is a peaceful and powerful way to bring it to the attention of those in charge. The collective power of names on a petition can be enough to instigate positive change. It's an easy way to get involved and help make the world feel less sh*t – so get signing!

Write a letter

It takes just a little more thought and time than signing a petition, but writing a letter is another peaceful, positive and proactive step you can take to help instigate change. If there's a local or political issue that's getting under your skin, writing a letter to your local MP is a way of bringing it to their attention and getting your voice heard. And if you're feeling helpless in the face of human rights injustices, Amnesty International's Write for Rights campaign has helped save thousands of lives – simply by putting pressure on governments through the power of letter writing.

The power of protest

Joining (or organizing) a peaceful protest is a powerful way to both call for positive change and boost your mental health if you're struggling with anxiety over political, environmental or global issues. Taking part in a march, sit-in or other demonstration alongside other like-minded people can foster a sense of solidarity and community, which in itself can make the world feel that bit brighter. Peaceful protest and freedom of expression is a human right, so if you feel inspired to join the collective, make some noise and call for change alongside others. You've got this!

The health benefits of helping others

When you start giving back to the community, when you start recognizing others' needs and spending more time thinking about how to help those around you, you might discover some positive, personal pay-offs. Research shows that doing good deeds can result in a "helpers' high", as it stimulates your brain's reward centre and releases endorphins, which can increase feelings of happiness and boost self-esteem. What's more, helping others, forging connections within your community and seeing the positive results of your actions can help you see that perhaps everything hasn't gone to sh*t, after all. It's truly a win-win!

A Hopeful Future

"**H**ope is being able to see that there is light despite all of the darkness." This powerful quote from Archbishop Desmond Tutu is a reminder that hope exists even when life seems bleak. It's not about pretending bad things aren't happening, but about remaining optimistic that they will pass. In this chapter, we'll look at how to cultivate and maintain a more positive outlook, even through dark times, and how to remain hopeful for the future.

Reasons to feel hopeful

In a world where bad stories seem to constantly be breaking news, and where we can get lost in a never-ending cycle of doomscrolling on our phones, it's sometimes hard to stay positive. But remember, however loud and "in your face" the bad bits of life get, the good bits are still there, even if they're well hidden. So, if life feels sh*t and overwhelming right now, remember, there are always reasons to feel grateful, hopeful and positive – even something simple (yet at the same time, profound), like the sun rising, or your body working hard to keep you well. What small thing can you feel hopeful or positive about right now? Hold on to that as you go about the rest of your day.

Channelling realistic optimism

Remaining optimistic about the future is great – but blindly believing everything's going to turn out brilliantly, without taking any responsibility for this desired outcome, can often lead to disappointment. This is where realistic optimism comes in: feeling hopeful about the future while remaining conscious of the reality. Realistic optimism is about recognizing that there may be challenges ahead that will require some forward planning and navigation. It's a mindset that keeps you accountable for your own growth and limitations and steers you away from that "toxic positivity" realm, which tries to deny the occurrence of challenging circumstances.

Hope vs happiness

Happiness and hope don't always coexist. You don't need to feel joyfully happy in order to feel hopeful – you just need to stay open to the possibility of positive change. And change can always happen. We know this, because so many things – from the weather to our emotions – are in constant flux. Of course, happiness can often spring from feelings of hope, where hope is a positive state of mind in and of itself: if you can shine the light of hope into a dark situation, then you are bringing a little brightness, positivity and even joy to a difficult situation. So, if you feel like everything's gone to sh*t and happiness isn't an emotion you currently feel able to channel, try focusing on hope instead.

Find your happiness

Remember, there isn't a finite amount of happiness, luck or love in the world. Just because someone you know has recently found the love of their life, bought their dream home, bagged an exciting new job, announced a pregnancy, is jetting off on a round-the-world trip, or (insert any other event that you quite fancy for yourself), it doesn't now mean there's less chance that this exciting thing will happen for you.

OK, so this might seem obvious, but it's worth repeating (and remembering), because so often, on hearing someone else's good news, however happy you are for them it can

also leave you wondering, "When's it going to be my turn?".

It's important to note that this is a completely normal reaction – we've probably all felt it at some point or other in our lives. But it doesn't mean there are now fewer chances left for you.

There is infinite happiness in this world, so never lose hope that you'll get your big break and, equally, never leave everything to chance: what small steps can you take to increase the potential of your success? Can you write out a plan, apply for that new position or start saving for a dream holiday? Self-belief is vital, but putting in the work is just as important.

Practise radical acceptance

If you often find yourself trapped in a cycle of suffering and struggle with feelings of hope or optimism, often feeling like everything's sh*t, you might find that radical acceptance helps.

While it has roots in Buddhism, radical acceptance is a core principle of dialectical behavioural therapy (DBT), and is based on the idea that the suffering you're experiencing didn't arise directly from the painful experience you're going through, but from your attachment to that painful experience.

If you regularly find yourself thinking, "This isn't fair", "I can't handle this", or "Why is this happening?" then it probably shows you're

not willing to accept that a difficult or painful thing is happening. Of course, accepting that things are sh*t can be difficult, and professional help from a qualified therapist can be a good idea if you're struggling with the concept.

Radical acceptance doesn't mean you endorse or agree with the difficult thing; it simply means that you accept you have no control over it – you understand you can't change the reality of this moment – and so you can be free to feel your emotions without an extra layer of resistance.

Radical acceptance can be helpful when going through bereavement, sudden change (such as a job loss) or a relationship breakdown and, in time, can leave space for hope and optimism.

Remember how far you've come

Although we can often feel like everything's gone to sh*t, this mindset overlooks all the effort we've put in so far to making things less sh*t. Take a moment to reflect back on all your past achievements and successes. Often, we get so caught up in striving for the next thing, and the next, that we forget to acknowledge all of the steps that we've successfully accomplished already.

What did you used to hope and wish would happen for you that you've since achieved? Perhaps you passed an exam, succeeded in a job interview, were brave enough to go on a first date after previous heartache, wrote the

first draft of that novel, made a new friend, navigated a divorce or took an evening class. All of these things, and the others you've brought to mind, are worthy of celebration and praise. Go you!

It's so easy to dismiss the bravery, focus and determination it took to do things we've already done, so for a moment, congratulate yourself for everything you've already achieved, and feel grateful for the fact you took those steps. Sometimes, acknowledging how far you've come is a wonderful gateway into renewed hope and positivity for the future.

Remember where you're headed

Always remember, however difficult life might seem – however low, anxious, hurt or stressed you're feeling – you have the power to change your life, right now.

That might seem like a big, sweeping statement, but it's true. By implementing tiny changes today, such as starting a journal to untangle your thoughts, taking a short daily walk and doing a 10-minute meditation before bed, you can start to cultivate the mindset you need to feel happier, more positive and more hopeful for the future. Just because you feel like everything's gone to sh*t in this present moment, it doesn't mean the future's going to be sh*t too.

Look back over the last chapter: which self-care tips might you be able to integrate into your life immediately? Could you drink a glass of water (see page 83), make yourself a healthy lunch (see page 84) and head out to pick yourself up a little treat (it doesn't have to be big, as you'll see on page 91)?

How can you start to embody "future you" right now? How can you begin to live as though what you want is already a reality? By making small changes to your day-to-day life, as well as truly inhabiting the state of mind you wish to achieve, you have the power to transform your headspace and start living the life you deserve.

Switch up the way you view uncertainty

Feeling uncertain about the future can lead to nervousness and anxiety. But did you know that anxiety can have the same effect on your body as excitement? (Think about it: butterflies in your tummy, an elevated heart rate, racing thoughts...) So, if you're feeling uncertain about the future, why not try to reframe this feeling as excitement? The butterflies could be anticipation of the various possibilities that could arise. Instead of worrying about what might go wrong, try focusing instead on what might go right. After all, uncertainty isn't necessarily bad: if you don't know what's to come, why not channel those feelings into excitement and hope for positive outcomes?

Make "looking forward to..." lists

Make a list of all the things you're looking forward to today: your morning coffee, knowing you get to hug a loved one, reading a chapter of your book, and so on. Now, make a list of all the things you're looking forward to this week – perhaps going for a morning run or having dinner with a friend. Now, make a list of all the things you're looking forward to this year: a family reunion, a holiday, a protest march you're attending, and so on. Keep referring to your lists whenever you need hope and optimism, and make new lists whenever you fancy a pick-me-up! Noting down things to look forward to can help you identify all the good in your life – everything has not actually gone to sh*t.

Trust that this shall pass

"This too shall pass" is a very well-known mantra – and for good reason: because life is cyclical and everything progresses, changes and evolves.

So, if you're currently stuck in a challenging time – if you're experiencing anxiety, low mood, grief, loss, pain, resentment, fear or any other difficult emotion – know that it won't last forever. It will pass, like a rain shower or a season. Simply knowing that you will come out the other end of this difficult time, after processing these emotions, can offer some relief and hope, even as you are navigating your way through it.

And of course, this goes for the good times too: good times also pass and more challenging times may be ahead. In this way, the mantra "This too shall pass" can help you to live fully in the moment, appreciating every good, happy and joyful thing that comes your way, and truly feeling grateful and thankful for it in the knowledge that it won't last forever.

Knowing that everything passes can help you to fully dive into each and every experience of your life – both the good and the bad – allowing you to feel everything deeply, while remaining aware that it will change.

Look for the good in people

For the most part, people are good. Not everyone, and not always, but mostly. People want to help. People will return your smile, or your glove that you dropped as you passed them, or the favour you did them. So, if life is getting you down right now and everything feels a bit sh*t, pay closer attention to these little acts of goodness – it might just restore your hope and faith in humanity.

Seek out like-minded people

If you want to feel more hopeful and optimistic, try spending more time with the people who lift you up and make you feel good. You know the ones – the people who make you laugh, who celebrate your wins and who have your back. Hanging out with friends who honour your values, respect your boundaries and share your passions will help you to fill your life with joy, love and support. These are your people.

Limit your news consumption

If the first thing you do in the morning is reach for your phone and start doomscrolling through the news, consider whether this is a positive way to start the day. Of course, you probably want to keep up with current affairs, but constantly checking for news updates might be negatively impacting your mental health. Instead, set a time each day when you'll check the news (and a time limit of, say, 10 minutes), and then steer clear for the rest of the day, focusing instead on your present moment.

Curate your news feed

While current affairs news tends to focus on big, attention-grabbing stories, which sadly include global disasters and upheaval, there is actually a lot of good stuff going on out there, too. Try following some positive news feeds or sign up to receive positive news alerts and newsletters, which will help to give you a more balanced and uplifting view of the world. And if you do see an upsetting news story, is there any positive action you can take to help? Is there a fund you can donate to or a petition you can sign? Remember, action always beats apathy.

Practise positive visualizations

Even the most positive people struggle to feel optimistic sometimes. More often than not, joy, positivity and hope have to be cultivated and nurtured. If you've woken up in a less-than-hopeful mood, feeling a bit sh*t about your life or the state of the world, try a short visualization practice to help kickstart a more positive outlook. Close your eyes and imagine achieving a goal. Engage all your senses: what can you see, touch, hear, smell, even taste, as you achieve it? How does it feel to achieve it? Now step into your day as if it has already happened. Visualizing positive outcomes can enhance your confidence and self-esteem, which can improve your whole state of mind.

Harness the power of creativity

Numerous studies have found a link between creativity and mental well-being, because creative pursuits, such as painting or writing, can be powerful mindfulness tools, helping to draw your attention away from the things that are making you feel sh*t, and into the present moment. Creative pursuits can also be highly relaxing, helping you to unwind and process those difficult emotions. When it comes to creativity, the joy is in the doing, not in the outcome, so don't let thoughts of not being good enough hold you back: simply draw, paint, write, sculpt, crochet, or anything else that makes your heart sing, with abandon! Hopefully the process of creation will leave you feeling inspired, fulfilled and more optimistic.

Use negative emotions as signposts

If you're struggling with negative feelings and emotions, it's important not to berate yourself. All feelings have a purpose, so it's important not to simply slap a fake smile on your face and pretend your uncomfortable feelings aren't there.

Honour all of your feelings – tricky ones included – but instead of wallowing in them, try looking a little more closely at why the feelings are occurring. Might you be able to use your difficult emotions as a signpost for positive action?

For example, perhaps you're feeling jealous that someone you know has just bagged their dream job. Jealously can feel horrible, but what is it telling you? Might you be feeling stuck in a career rut? Has this person just bagged *your* dream job, hence the jealous feelings? Is it time for you to take the plunge and make a career move, too? Are you qualified to apply for a similar role? If not, could you sign up to an evening course to set yourself on your way?

By delving a little deeper, you might find you can set some positive steps in motion that could see you improving your life.

Be a cheerleader for others

If you want to be part of a world that feels more positive, optimistic and hopeful, it's time to project some of that energy out into the universe. Even if you're having a hard day, and even if things aren't going well for you just now, try to look for opportunities to compliment other people or congratulate them on their own achievements. Positivity can be contagious, so by exuding this energy for others, you'll likely start to feel more upbeat and hopeful yourself. In short, cheer for those around you and lift others up, and you'll be giving yourself a lift, too.

Gratitude and hope

We talked about the amazing health benefits of gratitude on page 70. But did you know that gratitude is also related to feelings of hopefulness in a big way? In fact, research shows that feeling grateful for things that have happened in the past can significantly increase our feelings of hope for the future – yet another great reason to reflect on all the good things in your life and note them down in your journal. Let your present gratitude inspire hope for a more positive future.

Celebrate the small stuff

If you're struggling to find things to feel positive about, and most things you call to mind are, well, a bit sh*t, you might not be thinking *small* enough.

So often, we only give ourselves credit when we feel we've accomplished something we consider to be "big", such as getting that promotion or new job. But the truth is, there's so much else we achieve each and every day that we could (and should) be celebrating!

Focusing on "smaller" wins will give you a series of small mood boosts throughout the day, and studies show that people who celebrate their small achievements end up

with increased feelings of motivation and positivity. So, start giving yourself credit for the small stuff!

From making your bed in the morning and eating a nutritious breakfast, to ticking off a task on your to-do list, reading a chapter of your book, putting a new boundary in place to protect your mental health, completing an act of self-care, doing some exercise, tidying a room or simply making it through a tough day, there is so much you have to feel proud of.

What have you done today that could be celebrated?

Look to inspirational people

If you're feeling low about the state of the world and wondering how you can possibly remain hopeful in the face of social injustices or environmental concerns, take a moment to look at those around you who are working to make a difference. It might be someone in a position of leadership, or an activist group, or even someone you know personally who is quietly getting on with positively impacting their little corner of the neighbourhood.

Take a moment to consider what they're doing. How are they remaining hopeful? (Hint: if they're taking action to fight for something

they believe in, then they're feeling hopeful for the future, because without hope, they wouldn't act. Without believing their actions might make a difference, they would simply give up.)

You can start taking action too, by volunteering for an important cause (see page 98), signing petitions (see page 104), marching in protest (see page 106) or sending letters (see page 105). Always remember that inspirational people are generally taking positive action, and action equals hope.

Hope for the future

Yes, there's a lot of bleak news out there – but it's definitely not all doom and gloom! If you want some reasons to feel hopeful about the future, consider the following:

* Single-use plastic bans have come into effect in many countries across the globe, including Bangladesh, France, the UK and Kenya, reducing plastic pollution and also the demand for plastic production, which contributes to climate change.

* Solar energy is forecasted to be the world's leading energy source by 2027.

* The hole in the ozone layer is healing, with studies showing it's on track to be completely restored within four decades.

* After they were destroyed by a tropical cyclone in 2016, coral reefs are now alive and well again in Fiji.

* The Indian rhino population now exceeds 4,000. When records began, there were fewer than 100, but conservation work and poaching bans are working.

* A new malaria vaccine has been found to be around 70 per cent effective at preventing malaria in children.

* Cancer survival rates have doubled over the past 40 years in the UK.

These are just a few reasons to remain hopeful for the future! What good-news stories can you find to add to these?

The health benefits of staying hopeful

Hope is a powerful and protective state of mind – and there are numerous mental and physical health benefits to prove it.

For a start, as you might expect, feeling hopeful has been shown to lessen feelings of stress and sadness. This is thought to be the case because those who feel hopeful adapt better in the face of adversity and feel greater life satisfaction.

But there's more: by cultivating a hopeful outlook, you might actually live longer! Research has found that those who remain hopeful are at lower risk of developing

cardiovascular disease and other chronic conditions, probably because they're more likely to take care of themselves with healthy eating, exercise and abstaining from smoking.

Is there some future challenge you've been worried about? How might you flip your outlook to become more hopeful? So, although things can sometimes feel like sh*t, channelling feelings of hope for the future can allow you to experience a happier, more optimistic present. Being hopeful will not only encourage you to create positive change, but it will also help you to enjoy a healthier here and now.

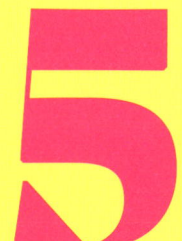

Seeking Help

Hopefully, the words in the previous chapters have offered you some solace and hope. They might have helped you see that, perhaps, not everything has gone to sh*t and, even if it has, it won't last forever and you will be OK. But, of course, you might feel you would benefit from additional support. If you're still struggling with worry, stress, low mood or other difficult emotions, you don't have to put up with feeling this sh*t – there is help available. The following pages will point you in the right direction.

Know there's no shame in needing help

If you've been feeling sh*t for a while, telling someone you're struggling can seem like a big deal. But remember, don't feel ashamed of asking for help. The mind is complex: anxiety, depression, grief, trauma and other mental and emotional responses can be all-consuming. One in four people experience mental health difficulties in developed countries, so you're not alone, and getting help from someone, whether it's a loved one or a professional, can be necessary to help you move on and feel better. There's no shame in needing help. Ever.

Open up to someone you trust

Often, one of the easiest initial ways to get help and support is to open up to someone you trust, such as a close friend or loved one. Often, telling someone you know well, and who cares about you, means you suddenly have an ally – someone who can offer comfort and support. It can also be a good way to practise speaking openly about your experiences, before making an appointment with a medical professional.

But, if the thought of looking them in the eye and blurting out that you've been feeling utterly sh*t recently makes you recoil in horror, don't panic. While this is a great way

to open up if you're feeling brave, it's not the only way.

If you're up for an in-person chat but don't fancy feeling like you are in the spotlight, going for a walk together can be easier, as you don't need to make eye contact if you're side by side. You could arrange a time to call them if you'd like a two-way chat but being face to face feels scary. Or talking via texts or messages is a good option, as it gives you time to think about what you want to say.

If you're worried your loved one won't know what to say or how to help, let them know that simply listening to you and being there for you is enough – sometimes, just having someone else hear your struggles, sympathize and let you speak your truth can help you to determine what it is that's bothering you and what other steps you could take to help yourself.

Use helplines or peer support

If you'd rather remain anonymous or you don't feel a loved one would be able to offer the support you need, calling a helpline or reaching out for peer support are great options.

HELPLINES

These will connect you with a trained specialist or volunteer who will listen impartially, without judgement, giving you a safe space to talk through your worries, concerns or problems. They may offer gentle prompts to help you explore your feelings more deeply, but they won't offer advice or opinions, and they won't make decisions for you. Many helpline volunteers will listen for as long

as you need, making them a good option if you're experiencing a crisis and want to talk until the immediacy of your thoughts have passed.

PEER SUPPORT

This involves people with lived experiences of a particular condition coming together to offer support and advice to each other. While there's no qualified "expert" offering advice, everyone's invited to share their experiences and insights, so it's great if you feel a sense of community would help you. Peer support can be accessed via your health professional, online, within your local community, or from student services if you're still in education.

Seek professional help

Everyone feels low sometimes. So, how are you supposed to know when to seek help? Accepting that your mental health problem goes deeper than simply "feeling a bit sh*t" can be hard, but don't put off seeking professional support if you're struggling. It's worth making an appointment with your doctor to chat about your mental health if:

* You are experiencing a persistent low mood, or feel "numb" or "empty"

* Your low mood or anxiety is interfering with your day-to-day life, such as your ability to work or interact with family or friends

* You're struggling to get out of bed in the mornings

* You think people would be better off if you weren't around

These feelings might feel like they're "you", and that they're here to stay – but it's not and they won't. With professional help, you can get back to feeling happy, hopeful and positive once more.

Determine what treatments are available

The first step to accessing professional support is to make an appointment with your doctor, who may refer you for further treatment, or to contact a private therapist directly, such as a psychologist or counsellor. The most common next step is talking therapy, such as CBT, counselling, or DBT, all of which have been shown to be effective in the treatment of mental health conditions, such as anxiety or depression.

Often, you'll need to commit to a series of sessions with a therapist, at the end of which you will hopefully have unravelled the difficult thoughts in your head and, in the case of CBT

and DBT, learned a set of coping strategies to help manage them in the future.

Medication is also available to help treat mental health conditions and may be offered alongside talking therapies. This is an option worth exploring with your doctor, as medication can help to ease the often debilitating symptoms of anxiety and depression, and it's often essential in the treatment of severe mental illnesses. Medication can make a profound difference, but if you're starting to feel better, don't stop taking them – it means they're doing their job! Always discuss potential dosage changes with your doctor.

Whichever treatment options your medical professional suggests, try to stay open-minded – they are there to support you and, hopefully with their help, you'll be feeling less sh*t very soon.

Access emergency support

If you experience a mental health crisis, accessing emergency support is vital. A mental health crisis could be:

* Experiencing suicidal feelings
* Having a panic attack
* Suffering from a manic episode
* Feeling like you might self-harm
* Any other time you feel your mental health is at breaking point

Emergency support isn't just about professional help – it's drawing on everyone you know who will help you at a time of crisis.

Creating an emergency plan can be helpful: who might you contact? Ask them if it's OK for you to call them if your mental health deteriorates. Also, keep the phone numbers of 24-hour helplines to hand: the support they offer during times of crisis can be lifesaving.

If you're in immediate danger – for example, if you've harmed yourself, have attempted suicide or are considering doing so – you should go to hospital or call an ambulance if you need to, call a helpline (you can explore various charities' services and find their helplines by visiting the websites listed on page 156), contact your local crisis team, or make an emergency appointment with your doctor.

Whatever you do, seek help. You are so valued, and life won't always feel this sh*t – honestly.

Conclusion

Even if you've been feeling like everything's gone to sh*t recently, hopefully these words have offered you some comfort, reassurance and hope. Low moments are inevitable – they're as much a part of life as the good bits – but they can feel super uncomfortable and upsetting. So next time you encounter a low point, where life feels sh*t and worries threaten to engulf your mind, flick back through these pages: remind yourself you're not alone, try out a few self-care tips and

reread a few reasons to feel hopeful. Being kind to yourself is important when things feel like they've gone wrong – doing so can help you navigate sh*t times more easily and quickly, and it can leave you feeling more resilient and able to appreciate the joys of life when the good bits come back round. And trust us, they will... so get stuck back into living your best life. Just because something's gone to sh*t, it doesn't mean everything has to. You've got this!

Resources

BOOKS

Fearne Cotton, *Bigger Than Us* (2022): Spiritual lessons for everyday happiness

Glenn Doyle, *Untamed* (2020): A wake-up call to stop pleasing other people, and instead start living your one true unique life

Matt Haig, *The Comfort Book* (2022): A collection of consolations learned in hard times

CHARITIES

Anxiety UK: This charity provides information, support and understanding for those living with anxiety disorders. anxiety.org.uk (UK)

Beat: This eating disorder charity helps to guide and support those with eating disorders, as well as their loved ones. beateatingdisorders.org.uk (UK)

CALM: The Campaign Against Living Miserably (CALM) is leading a movement against male suicide. thecalmzone.net (UK)

Mind: This mental health charity offers support and advice to help empower anyone experiencing a mental health problem. mind.org.uk (UK)

Samaritans: A 24-hour, free, confidential helpline, to support you whatever you're going through. samaritans.org; 116 123; jo@samaritans.org / jo@samaritans.ie (UK)

Anxiety & Depression Association of America: Education, training and research for anxiety, depression and related disorders. adaa.org (USA)

Freedom From Fear: A national non-profit mental health advocacy organization, helping to positively impact the lives of all those affected by anxiety, depression and related disorders. freedomfromfear.org (USA)

Mental Health America: Promoting the overall mental health of all Americans. mhanational.org (USA)

Mental Health Foundation: A non-profit charitable organization specialising in mental health awareness, education, suicide prevention and addiction. mentalhealthfoundation.org (USA)

National Suicide Prevention Line: 24/7 free, confidential support for those in distress, as well as crisis resources for loved ones. suicidepreventionlifeline.org; 1-800-273-8255 (USA)

PODCASTS

Bryony Gordon's Mad World: Intimate conversations about getting unwell... and then getting better

Griefcast **hosted by Cariad Lloyd:** Examining the human experience of grief

Happy Place **hosted by Fearne Cotton:** Conversations with inspirational people about life, loss and everything in between

Open **with Emma Campbell:** Open-hearted conversations about life's challenges, including both the messy and magical bits

Ten Percent Happier **hosted by Dan Harris:** Learn how to make your life better, through mindfulness and meditation techniques

Unlocking Us **with Brené Brown:** Unlocking the deeply human part of who we are, so that we can live and love more courageously

We Can Do Hard Things **hosted by Glenn Doyle, Abby Wambach and Amanda Doyle:** Getting through the hard things together, through open, enlightening conversations

IT'S OK TO FEEL SH*T (SOMETIMES)

Kind Words and Practical Advice For When You're Feeling Low

Sam Cooper

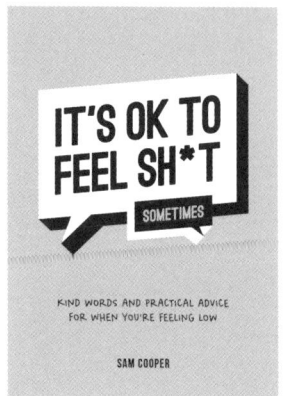

Hardback

ISBN: 978-1-80007-703-4

Packed with kind words and thoughtful advice, this informative guide is here to help you make sense of your feelings. With a breakdown of the most common causes of low mood, from work-related stress to clinical depression, this book teaches you how to recognize these issues and provides helpful tips on how to cope with them.